HEALTHY FOOD BOOK

DETOX DIET FOR LONG TERM HEALTH

HEALTHY FOOD BOOK

DETOX DIET FOR LONG TERM HEALTH

By

Shelly Jenkins, BSN RN

HEALTHY FOOD BOOK

DETOX DIET FOR LONG TERM HEALTH

Copyright © 2017 Shelly Jenkins, BSN, RN

ISBN-13:9781545282076

ISBN-10:1545282072

Printed in the United States of America

Kingdom Consulting Publishing
Columbus, OH

After you read this book if you feel like I've provided you with quality content and valuable information would you do me a HUGE favor please? I would appreciate it if you would write me a great five-star customer review for this book on Amazon. Hopefully our paths will cross at some point in our lives and we can meet each other in person. I pray that you will be blessed with perfect health, abundant wealth and never-ending happiness! Feel free to contact me at the email address below. God bless you!

EMAIL:

Shellyjenkins13@gmail.com

DEDICATION

To Stephanie, Aniya and Aaron,
my inspiration.

TABLE OF CONTENTS:

Introduction

Appendix

Introduction

I was just about to give up. I had been on a food plan for 7 years by this point. Abstaining from a lot of food by this time. Had tried doctors and a number of things to lose weight (including exercise) before even that. I managed to keep the weight off during the last stint. Of course I tried starving it off but then I would play catch up.

I had physical problems with my body for years: stomach aches and gas, acid reflex, heartburn, and skin breakouts. My stomach acid was like a three alarm fire (especially when I was pregnant). I had back pain, knee pain and joint stiffness. I had more problems than that but I will discuss those later.

A lady came into this meeting I was attending and I knew when I saw her that she was different. She seemed clear headed and serene. I had to find out how she achieved this? When I went to look up her source I found people who had been hospitalized (treatment) because their problems had gotten so bad.

When it all boiled down, the final question I had to answer was "I'm I willing to stop eating addictive foods? Addictive foods?? My response was "just tell me what they are and I can do it."

I was told that I could not stabilize my situation if I were not going to do a thorough job of it. And I was also told that I needed to make a decision to permanently change or go back to being completely out of control with food.

So I made the decision to try because I know I was getting nowhere FAST. I didn't want to gain back all the weight I had lost, which was over 300 -350 pounds during my lifetime. I was given some guidelines and principles to follow. Then a list of food chemicals that I could no longer eat. Lastly, a plan for eating which if used would give me a daily reprieve and help me to eat for good nourishment and general surrender. I had learned that success usually comes after taking some suggestions.

So this is my journey on which I embarked. I hope that it will help someone change their life as it has helped me.

Chapter One

Preparing for a New Life

What you will need:

One large heavy garbage bag

The first thing I did was to evaluate what was in my house. If it was not going to be good for my new life style of nutritious healthy eating and being free it had to be thrown out.

I walked over to my kitchen cupboards and opened them up. Everything that was on my list of food that I could no longer have would be placed in the center of the kitchen table. I began to read labels, one item after another. If it passed, (meaning there were no ingredient in them that was on my list of chemicals) it went back in the cabinet, if it did not it went to the table. I went through all cabinets and read all labels on all foods. Then I opened the refrigerator and did the same. I even included spices. Anything "contaminated" went to the kitchen table. About half of the food in my house could no longer be used.   Now wonder I was still having trouble I thought.

All the foods that were on my table went into a large heavy garbage bag. This bag was taken out to the trash. Upon coming back to my house I felt this incredible feeling of safeness. I knew that from now on my house would be a safe place for me to live and eat. That was a good feeling.

Next, since my cupboards and refrigerator was pretty bare, I took soap and water and cleaned out my cabinets from crumbs and my refrigerator from spilled foods. I made this a deep cleaning since I knew I would be organizing and starting new. I washed all dishes and even organized them too. If they were old or I was no longer using them, I put them in a box for donations. I got out my place mats and napkins and organized them too (only keeping what I enjoyed using) and placed the remaining one's in for donations. Now I was ready for Step Two.

Here is the Food Plan I used:

<u>Breakfast 7am</u>
1 Protein
1 Grain
1 Fruit
1 Dairy

<u>Lunch 11:00 am</u>
1 Protein
1 Raw Vegetable
1 Cooked Vegetable
½ oil

<u>Dinner 4:00 pm</u>
1 Protein

1 Grain
1 Raw Vegetable
1 Cooked Vegetable
½ oil

Bedtime Half Meal 8:00 pm
1 Fruit
1 Dairy or 2 oz Protein

Men: Add 1 fruit or 1 grain, or 1 starchy vegetable. 2 Oil servings. Men need to add two ounces of fish or poultry or one ounce of red meat at each meal to the amounts shown on the list. At lunch, men also add a serving of one of the following: a fruit, a grain, or a starchy vegetable.

Meal Times

Lunch (4 hours after breakfast)

Dinner (5 hours after lunch)

Bedtime Half Meal (4 hours after dinner)

Chapter Two

Grocery Shopping and Food Preparation

Now it was time to get some food in the house. I took a friend the first time to help me read labels. They will have to have the chemical list so that they will know what foods you are trying to avoid.

I had with me my list of foods that I could eat and those items I would need for my first few days. I did not do too much grocery shopping that first day to keep from being overwhelmed. It was easier to go back if necessary. I also took a list of spices I didn't want to forget to buy.

Once I got home, I put up all my food and chopped up some of the vegetables for salads and placed them in storage containers. I lined items up by categories i.e. all grains went together, canned beans together. In the refrigerator I did the same. Fruits in once section and vegetables on another shelf in another section. Liquids together and dairy together. I wanted to be organize especially when I went to look and see what I had to plan the next day's meals. It is also helpful when you're running out of groceries and have to make your grocery list. It's frustrating to not have what you need for a meal once you get home.

Next I wrote down what I was going to eat for the next day. I make my plan clear and concise so that I will not miss any items for a meal. I list my proteins first, then my grain, then my fruit and then my dairy for breakfast. If it is my lunch and dinner I list my proteins first and then my grain, then any vegetables I am going to eat. First listing cooked vegetables then raw vegetables. At the end of the day I have a small meal so I don't have to go too long until breakfast. This is also to get in another protein and fruit serving. I have six serving of fruit and vegetables daily. A day of a planned meal looks like this:

Breakfast 7am
2 eggs
1 cup of oatmeal
I cup of mandarin oranges
1 cup of 1% milk

Lunch 11:30 am
4 oz. Tuna
1 cup chopped onions, bell peppers, cilantro and tomatoes
I cup of green salad
½ tbsp. salad dressing (oil)

Dinner
I cup black beans
1 cup brown rice
1 cup roasted vegetables
1 cup of green salad
½ tbsp. salad dressing (oil)

Bedtime Half Meal
1 cup watermelon
½ cup of ricotta cheese

I use the same plan each day just changing the food choices. I became very regimented by memorizing and following this each day. It gets easier as you keep doing this day in and day out.

Chapter Three
Organization

Since I knew my kitchen needed to be well stocked, I decided to get some new items to make food preparation easier. This is my complete list.

My Kitchen Items:

Food Scale

Measuring cups

Measuring spoons

Rice cooker

Small toaster oven

Vegetable slicer

A good cutting knife or cleaver

Storage containers

Towels and dishcloths

A Small Salad Dressing Container

A travel tote with a long strap

Whatever you have you can start with but as you go along start to pick up these items. This will help you to make food prep much easier and organized later. The items on the top of the list for weighing and measuring food is imperative. Later I purchased anything I thought would help me to slice or dice or store or carry for lunch. Some of those items are a tote container with strap for lunches and a large cooler with rolling wheels for out of town travel. Having these items makes it easy to have food whenever you need it. I didn't want to have an excuse to be without food and make a decision to eat out. Eating out generally means not knowing what is used to prepare the food. I was not strong enough to make those decision especially when I was hungry. It doesn't take much for it to fall apart quickly.

Chapter Four

Food Guidelines
And Starting the Plan

Now was the time for setting my guidelines for my new lifestyle. I use the following guidelines for health and nutrition.

1. I make sure I read all labels so I know what is in everything I am eating. I don't assume what is in an item. This is to guard my body against eating anything with the chemicals I have detoxed from. If I can't read it, then I don't really know what is

in it. Especially when eating outside of home. I rarely eat out. I look for the **ingredient section** of the label. Advertisement on the front of the containers are misleading! Terms like sugar free on a front label does not mean that the company who manufactured this product did not add sugar in another form.

2. I **weigh and measure** all of my food and I always abide by the food portions at all times. I was always eating more than a portion share in my bingeing episodes so this is important. I never

feel stuffed now due to over eating at a meal.

3. I only eat "can have foods" that is listed on my new food plan. I look for hidden ingredients on the packaging, including spices and salt.

4. I plan ahead by writing down what I will eat. This way I am organized and not vague about what I am doing with food on a daily basis. If I don't plan to succeed I am planning to fail.

5. I space out my meals so that they are not too close together and I am not going for long periods of

time without eating. That does happened since you lose cravings and your appetite. I eat bout every 4-5 hours. I don't go too long in between meals because it sets me up for binge eating later that day. It is also important so that later in the day you do not have a large amount of food to eat in a short period of time.

6. I change or rotate my food by not eating the same thing all the time. I need to get a variety of food for their nutrients.

7. I don't drink caffeine, or sugar sweeteners (of any

kind), alcohol, and diet sodas. These chemicals have sugar and cause cravings!

8. I eat frozen or fresh vegetables. Fresh is best. Essentially eating nothing that is processed. Good foods that are wholesome. A list is provided in the index.

9. I weigh myself the first day of the month.

10. I don't eat between meals. But I can have non caloric drinks, especially plenty of water between meals.

The next phase is when you start eating by the plan. Everyday it's the same plan but each day it's different food choices. This is what is going to make a difference in your life from this time forward.

As I began to detox by abstaining from the addictive chemicals **and** sticking to the food plan, my initial reaction physically to the regiment was a very strong headache that I could feel throughout my brain! The intensity let me know how significantly these chemicals effect our brains. It was a throbbing sensation, as if there was a feeling of insult to brain tissue. This went on for about 4 days. It was intense enough that I had to rest in a room with low lighting most of the day. You may not be in as deep as I was so don't let this scare you.

Also as time went on I began to get weaker and was not able to do a lot of physical activity. I suddenly realized that my body was so used to synthetic energy from processed foods for fuel that it did not know how to respond yet. It didn't know what to do without its drugs! It didn't even know what to do with whole foods! It scrambled.... It was as if I were not eating at all! As my body started to heal, which initially was a few weeks, it started to take up and utilize the food from the new food plan. So I started to experience spurts of new energy that were quit strong. They did not last long but it would feel like I could run around all day. I would forget what was happening and plan many things to do in my schedule, then get out there during the day and run completely out of energy! Had to literally crawl back home, lol. So I learned to be wise and take it easy the first two months because of this problem. I guess it was hard to believe how serious this all was, providing energy to my body through food. I now know that this problems is BIOCHEMICAL. Eventually the energy spurts lasted longer until my body healed. But it was unpredictable. After that I could exercise with the young people, run circles around them and not be sweating like them in my line dancing class. It was great to see how efficient my body would now run on this new "fuel" plan. I knew I was on the right track. I couldn't help but wonder how much better my health would be since this was such a drastic change from my old life style. A positive change.

Chapter Five

Life After Detox from Addictive Foods

I continued eating on the plan daily. It was tedious preparing meals daily with the weighing and measuring of food. So it became practical to start doing several servings at a time. Even cooking enough for several meals at a time. This is called batch cooking. I would cook a pot of brown rice and then weigh and measure the whole container and refrigerate or freeze it, depending on how soon I planned on using it. As I continued to practice daily, it began to get easier and I could get a meal ready in about 10 minutes. Sometimes I would take a Saturday morning and do this so my week would go smoothly. Chopping up vegetable and putting them in containers. For salad, I would pre-make them, assembling several of them at a time with all the added veggies (cherry tomatoes, cucumbers, shredded carrots, mushrooms and onion) of whatever I wanted on my salad. Then all I would have to do is add the dressing. I found that my biggest problem with food was eating my vegetables. I was really not accustom to eating a lot of them in the first place. Now I know that they contain minerals that are part of the 90 essential nutrients required for my body. Having salad made ahead of time lessened my tendency to make excuses not to eat them. Eventually, opening the refrigerator and seeing it organized and clean was quite an experience but it was so nice to know I could reach in and pull out containers with my meal prepared, heat and eat. I wished that I could have been this organized before because I could have saved a lot of time.

I started to notice some very encouraging results from being on the food plan for a longer period of time. I started to sleep soundly every night (within about a month). Not even waking up for a bathroom break. I would have panic attack, when I drive. All of a sudden I would get a thought and then the fear would grow, from out of nowhere. I would have to fight that fear while driving on the freeway and that was very scary. Sometimes I thought I was just going to jump out of my skin. It would cause me to step on the break to stop the car, but you can't do that on the freeway. One day I realized I was no longer struggling with it because my panic attacks subsided. Today, I can't even induce them!

My weight started to come down without delay. Especially that stubborn last 15 lbs. It was gradual but it was steady. No plateaus. When I reached my goal weight I noticed the weight loss did not stop. When my cousin said, you're melting away on me, I realized I needed to look at how far down the scale I should go. I had never been able to get the "final frontier" (15lbs) of weight off.

I eventually had to start a maintenance plan, and you will too (included in the appendix), which involves adding food back into the food plan in a gradual way. This is related to another facet of my weight lose problem, what to do after the weight comes off?? This was critical because my life pattern with my weigh was to lose it then gain it back. I could get it off but not keep it off. Up and down and up and down.

A lot of my fear about weight loss was about gaining it back. I lived in such fear! Subconsciously, I always planned to go back to my old habits and "eat like I want too". But that was no longer an option now. Besides, I had never got to the point of looking at this eating problem as something to continue walking out or should I say "walking in". I was in this for the long haul and quite frankly I was sick of the rollercoaster ride.

This time I wanted to know how to do it right. I wanted to know how to transition into a new life of maintenance, a life now without constant weight gain, misery, emotional pain, ridicule, obesity, fat people's clothes, and poor health. I wanted to be able to go into the "5, 7, 9 Shop" for God's sake!!! Most of all, since I finally found the successful way to lose weight (detox, **then** start a food plan so there are no craving to fight) I did not want to contaminate my body and I did not want to go through detox again. Detoxing was no picnic (but it was necessary). My body was clean and I was really enjoying that experience.

Before detoxing I had found two particular problems I had with my health that were food related. One was lactose intolerance and the other was wheat intolerance. These health problems only had one simple solution, to abstain. Once I quit drinking milk containing lactose, I was shocked to find out that constant low level GI upset and bouts with gas and heart burn and acid reflex began to dissipate. I didn't know a person could feel so good.

Abstaining from wheat initially came purely by accident. When I first moved to this city, I found a group that did West African dancing. I really loved it but my left knee started to give me trouble. I eventually had to go to the doctor who started giving me steroid injections directly into the knee area. The injections also contained an anesthetic to calm down the pain. But the doctor told me this would not be effective after a while. They took x-rays only to find that I had a torn ACL that was from an old injury! Sometimes I could feel my knee was unstable and a few times the bones felt like they were rubbing together. This pain was so excruciating that I had to stop dancing.

One day this lady in a meeting was talking about how she had carried so much weight around being obese that she had worn out the cartilage in her knees and her bones were "rubbing together". I thought to myself "I know what that feels like". But then she said something odd. That she had abstained from wheat and that now she doesn't have any pain in her knees (even though the cartilage was still worn down)! That turned my head...I thought about what she said because it wasn't like she had surgery, she just abstained from wheat and the problem had been removed.

Well, I had to try this because I didn't want that pain anymore. It took 6-8 weeks but I notice that I went into the winter without any knee **or** joint pain for that matter. I was pleasantly surprised but yes MY ARTHRITIS pain was gone! Later, I found that when you eat wheat it breaks down into gluten and that deposits around the joints and causes the stiffness and arthritis pain. What a simple solution. I would have been facing knee replacement the doctor said and that would only last 10 year and would need another. I was still pretty young so I would have that to look forward too. I'm so glad I did not have to go that far to find a solution and I'm glad that surgery was not it. Today, it's nice to know what was wrong and to be eating foods that are good for me and not making me ill.

Chapter Six

Emotional Detox

Now I bet you didn't think about this part. Most people don't and this is why they fail at this whole area of life, I did. I failed at keeping the weight off, failed at staying on my food plan, failed at maintaining good health (I did have it at one time, childhood I think), failed at staying at one size of clothes in my closet, failed at feeling and being, you know, slim. Failed at looking in the mirror and saying "I'm happy with the way I look', failed at continuing to honor myself.

So I'm going to go over this part of my journey. Now most people don't just eat "out of control" for nothing. First I had to realize that I was obese because I had an eating problem, not a weight problem. Next, I had to realize that **food** was my real problem, which I'm so glad this knowledge started to sink in, really. Weight gain always mystified me, why did it go up and down?? But when you get this revelation under your belt you'll realize that the ball is in your court and that now you have your power back. Power to choose, the power to do something about the problem, FINALLY, lol.

Now, people tell you and doctors tell you have a weight problem, cause that's what they see, your obesity. They don't see you binge eating late at night because of your "problems" or your "anxiety" or your "cravings". They don't know you rather eat than talk to them. They just see your weight when you step out the front door in the morning. See, I didn't get it. What YOU didn't see wasn't happening I thought. I was like the last person to know, lol! I used to eat in private, you know close the doors and nobody knows what I'm REALLY eating not realizing that what I was eating wasn't really important....it was THAT I was eating! And eating and eating....cravings make you eat. They grab you by the collar and say "get in that kitchen and pick out something to eat". All you need to know is what. It's even a fast food chain motto, you know "it's what you CRAVE". I didn't know what cravings really meant, I just knew something was driving me to eat because when I went on a diet (when I was REALLY trying) I had to fight "them" to stay the course.

This was my first experience with not having the phenomenon of craving. I went to a doctor for weight loss. I sat in the waiting room, where they have the 5 lbs. blob of fat model on the shelf so you could actually see what the fat problem looks like. They called my name and I saw the doctor. He said I want to give you B12 injections because you are malnourished. Oow I thought, a magic shot!

Then he told me I want you to pick a diet that you will use (oh snap, I forgot about that): high fiber or low carb. Well, this was during a time that everybody was going on these high fiber kicks, so I didn't want to hear any more about it. I picked the low carb diet. Next he said something to get me motivated. "What if I asked you to walk around carrying my 50 lbs. box over there, all day (he pointed to it)? Now you can't set it down, you have to carry it all day." I looked at him like he was crazy and fell right in the trap by saying, "That's too heavy, I couldn't do that!" Well, that's what you are doing every day that you are overweight he responded. **Light bulb moment!** Okay, that helped. After that shot I went home and started the diet.

On the first day I fixed the food and ate it. Stay with me here, and sat down to watch TV. Now I usually don't just watch TV, I eat. I usually run to the kitchen during commercials and get back when the program starts, if I rush. So…when the commercial came I hopped right down and ran to the fridge, I ate some "diet food" and watched the rest of the program.

Day Two, I fixed the food and ate it. I sat down to watch TV. When the commercial came I hopped right down and went to the kitchen and opened the refrigerator, the clock was ticking so I had to grab something quick, but I couldn't remember what I came in there to eat. I scratched my head and said that's funny, what was I going to get? When I heard the program coming back on, I ran back to the TV a bit baffled about why I didn't get anything to eat, but I continued to enjoy my program. Then another commercial, I hopped right down and went to the kitchen but dog gone it, I couldn't remember what I had a taste for. That's strange I never had this problem before. I closed the fridge door and slowly walked back to the bedroom and continued to watch TV until my program was over.

Day three, I fixed the food and ate it. I went to the bedroom and started to watch TV. I watched a two hour movie without ever getting up. When it was over, I realized that I hadn't got up to get any food.

Matter of fact, I didn't even want anything. Wow, that's strange.

A week later I had fallen off the diet. Later in life, I realized that I "relapsed" out of habit, not cravings. It's emotional, once the chemicals were removed and the cravings have gone with them, I was just getting up and going to the kitchen out of **habit**. These were my binge foods (my friends) that give me emotional comfort. If I knew what it all meant I might not have introduced it back into my system and started the cycle all over again. And I would have understood why my system was starting to quiet down. It was because I was not having cravings anymore. I think I would have realized I was no longer helpless and was in charge of my appetite again (which was almost nil).

But I learned from the experience. A low carb diet means a "NO (artificial) SUGAR" diet. It's the SUGAR that makes me crave! Now the revelation about the chemical SUGAR was clear. They put it in **ALL** the food. No wonder everybody's woofing down the food! We can't help it because we can't fight it. Only abstaining from it gets the situation back under control. Only then do I have a choice about when and what I want to eat, emotionally.

Yes, the lights were now coming on. Now I had to face the fact that if I picked up my binge foods it was being done for a deeper reason, not physiologic or BIOCHEMICAL. I had to admit that some foods are my friends. They help me cope through life, they listen when I'm upset. Especially when I'm upset with other people, I take my anger out on myself because I can't do that to them (or so I thought). Yes, normal people don't have a relationship with food!

Then there is another problem I have. I use foods because they do have a biochemical effect, like pharmaceuticals. I used them for mood stabilizers (fats), antidepressants (wheat), tranquilizers and pain killers (flour), and uppers (sugar). Because I used them as medication for my feelings, this was now a journey of feeling again and coping with what I had not confronted before. Since this experience was new to me, I had to realize that I could do it but not overnight and not without a support system. I give one in the bibliography of this book. I also have a couple of friends that are in the same situation but are climbing out too. We support one another. Journaling is also a way to process my feelings. When I get it down on paper it seems to leave and then I can see it in black and white.

Another thing I had to look at was why I was so out of control and how could I do this to myself? I thought that it was odd that someone could treat themselves like this. I prayed and one day sitting in a meeting the answer came. I was having an out of body experience when it came to food. There was no way I could get away with that if I was still present in my body, I was disassociating. That explained it all to me. God told me that day, "Go back and get her". He was referring to the true me. The one who had got kicked to the curb when this whole thing started. I didn't quite know when that was or where I kicked her out but I knew He was right. So I began the emotional journey of turning around as if I had taken a long trip, like from California to the Midwest, and started looking for the true me.

If you have ever made that trip in a car you know there are hundreds and hundreds of miles to look. I thought "what if she was left in the desert or in the mountains somewhere". I was afraid because metaphorically speaking I didn't know if she was still alive and what condition I would find her in. This really sadden me but each day that I made the effort to look for her I began to heal and one day I realized that she was back. She needed help but she was still alive. It was good to feel again so today I don't take that for granted. I will take staying present in my body and feeling again any day. You know why? Because I can no longer get away with eating like that and not caring about what will happen to me. I can't do it and demoralize myself any longer. I have finally learned to love myself enough to care.

Chapter Seven

Spiritual Detox

Now this chapter may appear to have the implication that you are cleaning out your spirituality. But it's really about getting rid of the negative things that keep us separated from a higher source. For me this source is God and I realized that I couldn't have two things sitting on the throne of my heart. You can only have one master The Holy Bible says.

"No man can serve two masters: for either he will hate the one, and love the other; or else he will hold to one, and despise the other. You cannot serve God and mammon."

I believe this holds true to anything that is your master, not just money. And food certainly was ruling my life, honestly. Spirituality is about heart issues.

I think the change began when I was willing to get help in the first place. I had gotten beaten down pretty bad. As I mentioned in the introduction of this book I had lost and gained about 300-350 lbs. over my life time. I kept trying but didn't have the solution. And spiritually speaking I was not ready to completely surrender.

The health problems were the consequences that got my attention and made me become willing. Once it all started piling up on me and I couldn't take it anymore, then I became willing.

I didn't know what the chemicals hiding in the food we eat would do to me eventually. Today, I know it is "deceitful food". I know that's why God started showing me how to get out of that deep dark hole when I cried out enough. Today, I can't stand to see others unknowingly trapped in the prison like I was. That is my motivation for taking the time to write this book. So I hope someone will get the help they need from reading it.

Also there is nothing better than being reconnected to the best guidance you can ever have. My connection or **uplink** to God has been the greatest advantage I could have in life today. Without it, this is a big world to get lost in. The guidance from Him has been life changing and invaluable, better yet, priceless.

"When my father and my mother forsake me, He will lift me up.

Psalms 27:10

When I used the story about God telling me to go back to get my authentic self I realized the depth of His compassion for me. I would never have known that what I needed most was me. That was the greatest healing I have gotten in this area of my life and it has reached into other areas of my life by giving me confidence, self-esteem, self-love and purpose. It's a good feeling to look in the mirror and LIKE yourself and not HATE yourself.

Casting all your anxiety upon him, because he careth for you.

1 Peter 5:7.

Funny these words were on a little plaque that was given to me as a young girl and it hung

on the doorway of my bedroom
for many years. It now has
become an important truth in
my life and I have come to
believe it in my heart.

I know there are those who
do not believe in God and that
doesn't stop anything because
He believes in us. I believe that it
is good to know that when you
are ready, he is waiting. And if
you never become ready, he is
still waiting.

I must say this also that He
lowered the bar for me to step
over it. He didn't make it
impossible to reach Him. I just
had to ask.

Most importantly, Spirituality means getting rid of the negative thoughts that you can do this on your own and without help. I couldn't. It became painfully obvious to me that I did not have the power to combat this problem and I never will. Today, I have learned that that power comes from God and I don't have to understand it to operate in it. Because of this I don't even rely on failing because I'm not using my power now, I'm using His power so failure is no longer an option. When I become afraid that this won't keep working, I remind myself that I never started by using my own power anyway.

Then I relax again and let Him take over. I let go and let God be God. It's so much easier.

"....For he that cometh to God must believe that he is, and that he is a rewarder of them that (diligently) seek after him.

Hebrews 11:6

Chapter Eight

Keep It Going

Now that you have detoxed and see what life is like without the use of addictive food you should be as impressed as I was. Part of my motivation now is the fact that I feel better physically and emotionally because I have taken back control over my life, my weight, and my health. I was beginning to enjoy some real health benefits that didn't cost me surgery, medical expenses, and false hopes. This was real and all it cost me was discipline and the desire to quit eating the addictive chemicals!

I cannot say that this is easy, so I want to share with you how to keep it going. This MOMENTUM is very valuable. Once you started to feel clean and confident, don't let it slip away.

I learned to protect this abstinence by not people pleasing and allowing what others do to influence my health program. I realized that others would probably never believe in what I was doing but that I could not suffer for what they may be thinking. Sometimes people look at food as love and they will try to force it upon you. Others will get offended even though it has nothing to do with them. Still others will think you are crazy and entice you to join the human race again.

There will be many people eating around you all the time, all kinds of food THAT YOU USED TO EAT and quite frankly it gets really hard. But I had to learn new emotional strategies to cope with people to protect my new life style. Everything from eating before I go somewhere, bringing my own food or just declining the invitation. I have changed my house around to make it look like a restaurant (I put the kitchen table in front of my living room bay window) so I could enjoy looking out the window while eating. I set a very luxurious table so it feels like a restaurant when I sit down to eat and I don't have to tip the waitress! Remember this is a new way of life and that means that we are not turning back. Going forward means learning new and enjoyable ways to keep up the lifestyle that brings freedom. All it takes is creativity.

This is one mentality that I had to get rid of and that's diet mentality. That means thinking that once I have achieve my weight goal, I kick the plan to the curb and go back to my old way of living. The consequences are too scary to think about. Know that you have nothing to look forward to but a refund on your misery. And remember it is easier to stay on the plan than to detox and get back on the plan. So being committed and creative is key. Don't give up the first experience of abstinence because it is like a jewel. If you lose it, it will not be the same.

Another thing I feel is truly important is your overall purpose for doing this in the first place. Losing weight for most people will be their "vanity goal". Most people go on diets because of their vanity. They want to get their weight off but not change anything else. But that mindset will not keep you going for the long haul. You will find it to be very difficult to meet the challenges that discipline takes with your ego driving the car. When I realized this, it was a **light bulb moment**. I only came to this conclusion after I realized I **was** struggling. Then I knew that I had to have a more powerful reason to continue to motivate me. That reason is **MY HEALTH**. This is the kind of reason that my God could get behind. He will give me power to have and keep my health because I know He says it's His will.

If I look at eating now as how to have a natural cure to illness, for wellness and the blessing of walking in divine health, I will be enabled to do that. Gluttony is not God's will for my life.   The sacrifice of eating well means you will have health other people will never experience.

Today, I am not having the health problems I used to have and do not take the medications that most people are destined to take. This costs me less money and gives me peace of mind. As I discuss in my first book "Natural Cures for Perfect Health" I am in charge of my health through discipline and consecrating my body for the purposes of God. This one simple act brings big results and benefits.

If you can find others that are like minded, even one buddy to walk the path with you, it will be very helpful. Again, I have a given a resource at the end of the book to use. But this is a great new life and the results are awesome.

Last of all, the "food problem" in this country is growing at an alarming rate. Most adults are now obese (two-thirds) are overweight or obese and 1 in 20 extremely obese and so are the many children (14% of children ages 2 to 5 and 31%

ages 10-17) who inherit this problems from the adults who raise them.

Stay fast to your solution and remember that each day you keep working toward staying on your food plan, you are rinsing this problem out of your life. It will happen in stages. Your abstinent will increase by levels, so don't ever give up. Only those who give up fail. BE BLESSED!!

APPENDIX

Chemicals to Avoid

Ace-K

Acesulfe-K

(Sunette, Sweet and Safe, Sweet One)

Aguamiel

Alcohol, Alcoholic drinks

Alitame

Amasake

Artificial Sweeteners of any kind; Equal, Splenda, Sweet'n'low, SweetThing

NOTE: All artificial sweeteners are considered sugar.

Artificial Flavors (check with company)

Aspartame/NutraSweet

Barley Malt

Cane Juice

Caramel coloring

Concentrated fruit juice

Corn sweetener

Cyclamates

Date paste, syrup

Dextrin

Dried/dehydrated fruit

Evaporated cane juice (e.g., Florida Crystals)

Extracts

Fat substitutes (made from concentrated fruit paste)

Fructooligosaccharides (FOS)

Fruit flavoings (chck with company)

Fruit juice concentrate
Glucoamine/glucosamine

Glycerine

Honey (any type)

Jaggery

-ides, any additive with this suffix: monosodium glycerides, olyglycerides, saccharides (any), trisaccharides, diglycerides,, disaccharides, glycerides (any), monoglycerides, onosaccharides, etc.

Licorice Root Powder

"Light", "lite" or "low" sugar

Malted barley

Maltodextrines

Malts (any)

Molasses, black strap molasses

"Natural" sweeteners

Nectars

Neotame

-ol, any additive with this suffix: carbitol, glucitol, glycrol, glycol, hexitol, inversol, maltitol, mannitol, sorbitol, xylitol, etc.

Olestra (made from sucrose)

-ose, these additives with this suffix:colorose, dextrose,

fructose, galactose, glucose, lactose levulose, maltodextrose, maltose, mannose, polydextrose, polytose, ribose, sucralose, sucrose, tagatose, zylose.

Raisin juice, paste or syrup

Rich malt, sugar or syrup

Rice sweeteners

Saccharin, liquid saccharin

Sorghum

Splenda (Sucralose)

Stevia

Sucanat (evaporated cane juice)

Sucraryl

Sugars, any type: apple sugar, Barbados sugar, bark sugar, beet sugar, brown sugar (any grade), cane sugar, caramel sugars, confectioner's sugar, date sugar, grape sugar, invert sugar, milled sugar, "natural" sugar, powdered sugar, raw sugar, turbinado sugar, unrefined sugar, etc.

Sunenette/Sweet-One (Acesulfamek)

Syrups, any type: agave syrup, barley syrup, brown rice syrup, corn syrup, date syrup, high fructose corn syrup, maple syrup, raisin syrup, yinnie syrup (rice syrup), etc.

Vanillin

Whey (as an additive)

Xanthan gum

Types & forms of wheat:
Bran (if made from wheat)
Bulgar
Cracked wheat
Durum wheat
Gluten (wheat protein)
Kamut
Red wheat
Red spring wheat
Seitan (made from wheat
protein, gluten)
Semolina
Spelt
Triticale (a wheat/rye hybrid)
Wheat berries
Wheat bran
Wheat flakes

Wheat germ
Whole-grain wheat
Winter wheat

Foods I Can Eat

Protein

Note: Men: Eat 5 oz. of red meat and 6 oz. of fish or poultry

Beef	4 oz.
Chicken	4 oz.
Dried Beans	1 cup cooked
Eggs	2 medium
Fish	4 oz.
Hot Dogs (not sugar cured)	4 oz.
Lamb	4 oz.
Pork	4 oz.
Shellfish	4 oz.
Turkey	4 oz.

Veal	4 oz.
Vegetarian (Tofu, Tempeh)	6 oz. Protein

Vegetables 1 Cup

Artichoke

Asparagus

Bamboo Shoots

Beans (yellow or green)

Bok Choy

Beets

Broccoli

Brussel Sprouts

Cabbage

Carrots

Cauliflower

Celery

Chicory

Chinese Cabbage

Cucumber

Dill Pickles

Eggplant

Endive

Escarole

Greens*

Mushroom

Okra

Onions

Peppers

Pimentos

Radishes

Rhubarb

Romaine

Rutabaga

Sauerkraut

Snow Pea Pods

Spinach

Summer Squash

Swiss Chard

Tomatoes

Turnips

Vegetable Juice

Water Cress

*Beet, collard, dandelion, kale, all types of lettuce, mustard, any sprouts (no Wheat grass)

NOTE: Tomato juice or vegetable cocktail juice without sugar may be used as a cooked vegetable substitute. 1 cup juice=1 cup cooked vegetables.

Fruits

Apple	1 medium
Apple Juice	½ cup
Applesauce	½ cup
Apricots	3 medium
Berries	1 cup
Citrus Juice	1 cup

Cantaloupe	½ (6" dia.)
Cherries	1 cup
Cranberry Juice	1 cup
Fruit Cocktail	1 cup
Grapefruit	½ large
Grapes	1 cup
Honeydew	¼ (7" dia.)
Kiwi	3 small
Lemons, Limes	2 small, 1 large
Nectarines	2 small, 1 large
Orange	1 large
Peach	1 large
Pineapple	1 cup
Pineapple Juice	½ cup
Plums	3 medium

Prune Juice	½ cup
Tangerine	2 small
Watermelon	1 cup

Grains

1 cup of any of the following, measured after cooking:

Amaranth

Barley

Brown Rice

Buckwheat

Cereals: Puffed brown rice, puffed corn, puffed millet

Grits

Millet

Oat Bran*

Oatmeal +

Quinoa

3 Rice Cakes =1 serving

Cream of Rye

Rye

*(1/2 Cup raw=1 cup cooked)

+Non-wheat sugar-free dry cereal

Starchy Vegetables

Baked Potato (white)

1 small 6 oz.

Beans: Lima, Navy, all dried beans ½ cup cooked

Corn	1 medium
Mashed Potatoes (white)	
	½ cup
Mashed Yams	½ cup
Parsnips	½ cup
Peas, dried	½ cup
Peas, green	½ cup
Pumpkin	½ cup
Sweet Potato	1 small, 6 oz.
Squash*	½ cup

*Acorn, Butternut, Hubbard, Winter and Spaghetti Squash

Beverages

Suggested drinks are water, carbonated water, herbal tea, decaffeinated coffee or decaffeinated tea.

Clear soup (without sugar) is permitted before lunch or dinner.

Tomato juice or vegetable cocktail juice without sugar may be used as a cooked vegetable substitute. 1 cup juice = 1 cup cooked vegetables.

Please note: All diet sodas have artificial sweeteners, which are now known to create cravings similar to sugar.

Dairy

NOTE: Dairy may also be used as a protein.

Buttermilk	1 cup
Low-Fat or Non-Fat Ricotta Cheese	½ cup
Milk: Skim or 1%	1 cup
Low Fat Cottage Cheese	½ cup
Low or Non-Fat Yogurt	1 cup
Unsweetened Soy Beverage	1 cup

NOTE: If you are dairy sensitive, eliminate dairy and substitute 2 oz. of any type of protein.

Fats

Polyunsaturated oils are essential to good health. The fat requirement is normally divided between two or more meals.

Women require one fat serving per day and men require two.

Choose from the following:

Oil   1 tablespoon

Mayo   1 tablespoon

Margarine 1 tablespoon

Salad Dressing

                2 tablespoons

Condiments

Any spice or sauce that is sugar-free, alcohol-free or wheat-free including, but not limited to, mustard, tamari, salsa, non-fat yogurt, lemon juice, etc. Limit spice and condiment use to the levels recommended in recipes or no more than 1 teaspoon per day of any one spice and no more than two tablespoons per day of any one sauce.

Maintenance Plan

This is really simple, the idea here is to stop weight loss and stabilize it. Also remember, the idea is not to go back to old patterns of eating. This will also help if you're at your normal or ideal weight. Then you will not need to lose weight just get sanity. If you are underweight this will help you achieve an ideal weight too. It even helps if you have fast weight loss.

Step 1: Add a grain or a starch serving to lunch meal.

Step 2: Use 2 tablespoons of oil in a day.

Step 3: Eat another fruit serving during a meal.

Step 4: Add in 2 oz. of protein during a meal.

Step 5: Add a cup of raw vegetables to any meal.

You do not want to let the weight loss get out of hand so monitor it by changing from monthly weigh-ins to weekly weigh-ins.

More than 2 lbs. weight gain means you do not need this much food so go back to the level you just left. If you do not stop losing weight, keep adding foods according to the steps above by going back to step one again.

Prayer of Salvation

If you have not made a decision to become a citizen of the Kingdom of God, Jesus is the door, or the way, the truth and the life. Here is a simple prayer you can say to receive the gift (of salvation) that keeps on giving:

"Dear God, I want to be a part of your family. You said in Your Word that if I acknowledge that you raised Jesus from the dead, and that I accept Him as my Lord and Savior, I would be saved. So God, I now say that I believe You raised Jesus from the dead and that He is alive and well. I accept Him now as my personal Lord and Savior. I accept my salvation from sin right now.

I am now saved. Jesus is my Lord. Jesus is my Savior. Thank you, Father God, for forgiving me, saving me, and giving me eternal life with You. Amen!"

WELCOME TO THE KINGDOM OF GOD!

Please go to a bible believing church to be taught about the Kingdom and to learn the Word of God. It will transform your life.

Bibliography and Resources:

For information regarding the food plan presented in this book, visit this website:

www.foodaddictsanonymous.org

Sheppard, Kay. *From the First Bite*. Deerfield Beach, FL: Health Communications, Inc., 2000.

If you enjoyed reading this book, here's more books by the author:

1. Natural Cures for Perfect Health: Jesus Christ Will Cure You But the Doctor's Won't
http://amzn.to./2Dz23a0

2. Natural Cures for Perfect Health Workbook
http://amzn.to/2M3bwao

3. Health Food Book, Detox Diet for Long Term Health
http://amzn.to/2pdf536

4. God's Health Care System, Receiving Healing Health Stories From The Holy Bible

http://amzn.to/2CYociL

5. Aniya's Health and Food Book
http://amzn.to/2tnCi4b

6. Aaron's Preschool Book Fruits of the Spirit
http://amzn.to/2p4n5Hn

7. Aaron's Preschool Book For 3 Year Olds: A Little Boy's Adventures
http://amzn.to/2qzFgo5

8. Aaron and Aniya's Beginners Bible, A Children's First bible Book
http://amzn.to/2t5vCau

9. El Sistema de Salud de Dios, Dios Tiene su Propio Sistema que Funciona

http://amzn.to/2legDTF

10. ¡Curas Naturales Para Una Salud Perfecta! Jesucristo Lo Sanará, Pero los Médicos no

http://amzn.to/2M5Oroj

11. The End of Slavery: Free to be Healthy

http://amzn.to/2GXtl7o

About the Author

Shelly Jenkins is a native of Chicago, Illinois and has been a believer in Christ since young adulthood. An avid bible scholar and bachelors prepared registered nurse for more than 34 years, she has worked in a variety of nursing areas including Maternal Child Health, Nursing Education, and Child Welfare Services. A school nurse for over 13 years and legal nurse consultant, she has a passion for health, healing and wellness through a biblical perspective. As a natural health consultant, speaker and ordained minister, she aspires to educate people about the health care system of God so that they may experience true health. An artist in her spare time, she is a mother of two and a grandmother of four and is currently living in Columbus, Ohio.

Contact Information

Email:

shellyjenkins13@gmail.com

www.godshealthcaresystem.com

Podcasts

Check out my Podcasts!

God's Health Care System

*On the Free **Anchor** App for more of my teaching!*

NOTES